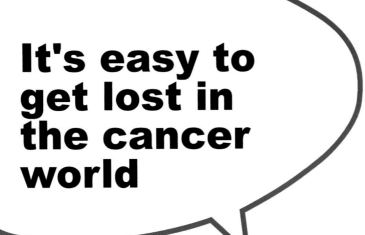

It's easy to get lost in the cancer world

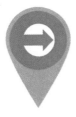

Let NCCN Guidelines for Patients® be your guide

✓ Step-by-step guides to the cancer care options likely to have the best results

✓ Based on treatment guidelines used by health care providers worldwide

✓ Designed to help you discuss cancer treatment with your doctors

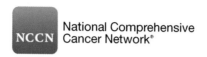

National Comprehensive Cancer Network®

NCCN Guidelines for Patients® are developed by the National Comprehensive Cancer Network® (NCCN®)

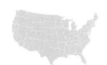

NCCN

✓ An alliance of leading cancer centers across the United States devoted to patient care, research, and education

Cancer centers that are part of NCCN:
NCCN.org/cancercenters

NCCN Clinical Practice Guidelines in Oncology (NCCN Guidelines®)

✓ Developed by experts from NCCN cancer centers using the latest research and years of experience

✓ For providers of cancer care all over the world

✓ Expert recommendations for cancer screening, diagnosis, and treatment

Free online at
NCCN.org/guidelines

NCCN Guidelines for Patients

✓ Present information from the NCCN Guidelines in an easy-to-learn format

✓ For people with cancer and those who support them

✓ Explain the cancer care options likely to have the best results

Free online at
NCCN.org/patientguidelines

These NCCN Guidelines for Patients are based on the NCCN Guidelines® for Management of Immunotherapy-Related Toxicities, Version 1.2022 – February 28, 2022.

NCCN Foundation seeks to support the millions of patients and their families affected by a cancer diagnosis by funding and distributing NCCN Guidelines for Patients. NCCN Foundation is also committed to advancing cancer treatment by funding the nation's promising doctors at the center of innovation in cancer research. For more details and the full library of patient and caregiver resources, visit NCCN.org/patients.

National Comprehensive Cancer Network (NCCN) / NCCN Foundation
3025 Chemical Road, Suite 100
Plymouth Meeting, PA 19462
215.690.0300

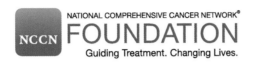

NATIONAL COMPREHENSIVE CANCER NETWORK®

NCCN FOUNDATION

Guiding Treatment. Changing Lives.

NCCN Guidelines for Patients are supported by funding from the NCCN Foundation®

To make a gift or learn more, please visit NCCNFoundation.org/donate
or e-mail PatientGuidelines@NCCN.org.

Sponsored by

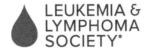

LEUKEMIA &
LYMPHOMA
SOCIETY®

The Leukemia & Lymphoma Society (LLS) is dedicated to developing better outcomes
for blood cancer patients and their families through research, education, support and
advocacy and is happy to have this comprehensive resource available to patients.
LLS.org/PatientSupport

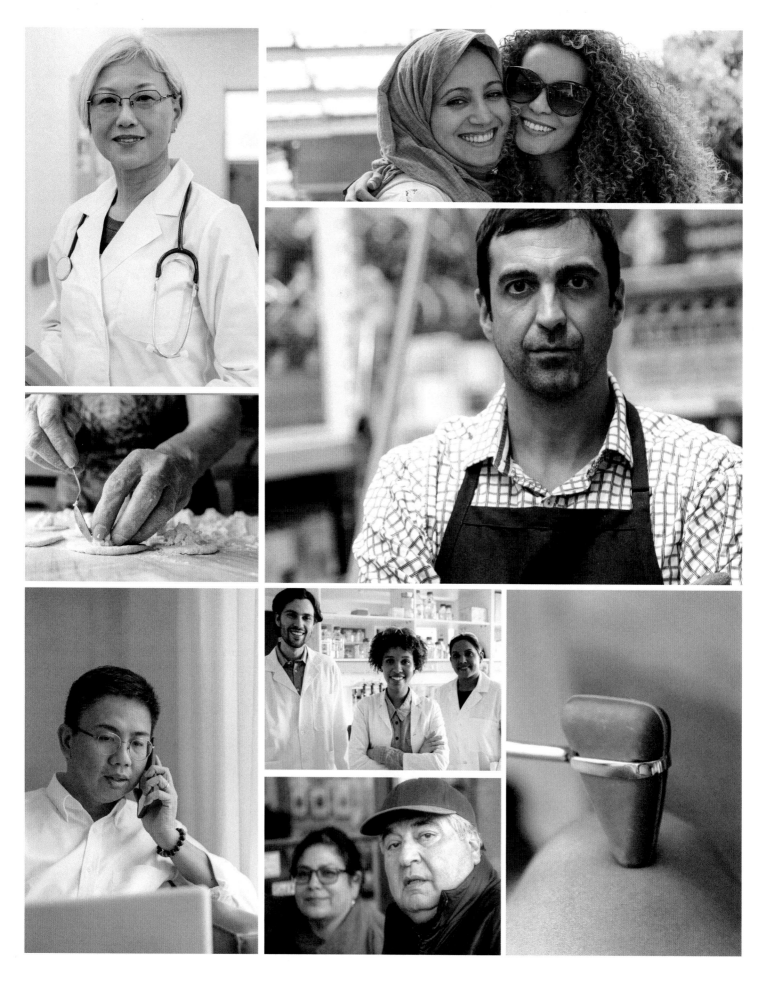

Contents

1

CAR T-cell therapy basics

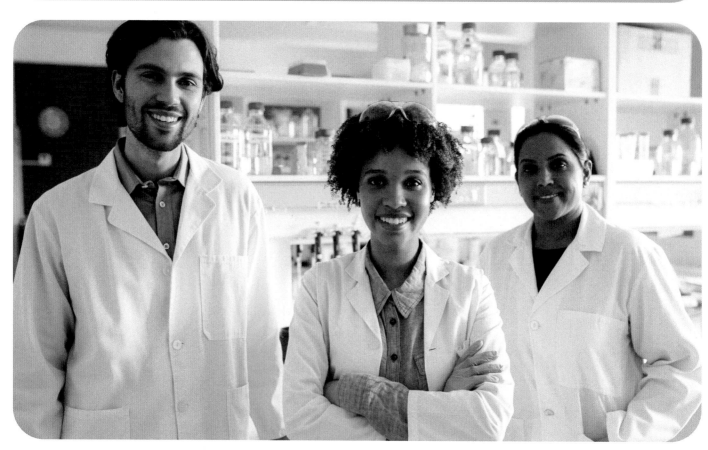

CAR T-cell therapy is a recent breakthrough in blood cancer treatment. Called a "living drug," CAR T is highly effective but can also be harsh. Severe and possibly life-threatening effects are possible.

What is CAR T-cell therapy?

CAR T-cell therapy is a type of immunotherapy. Immunotherapy uses the immune system to fight cancer. CAR T works by changing your own immune cells in a way that allows them to find and kill cancer cells.

CAR T is currently used to treat certain blood cancers that did not respond to other treatment, or that have come back after treatment. This includes some forms of lymphoma and leukemia, and multiple myeloma.

At this time there are 6 CAR T-cell therapies approved by the U.S. Food & Drug Administration (FDA) for cancer treatment:

> Tisagenlecleucel (Kymriah)

> Axicabtagene ciloleucel (Yescarta)

> Brexucabtagene autoleucel (Tecartus)

> Lisocabtagene maraleucel (Breyanzi)

> Idecabtagene vicleucel (Abecma)

> Ciltacabtagene autoleucel (Carvykti)

The first 4 listed therapies bind to a protein called CD19. CD19 is found on the surface of some leukemia cells and most B-cell lymphoma cells. The last 2 listed are used to treat multiple myeloma. Multiple myeloma is a cancer of plasma cells. These therapies target B-cell maturation antigen (BCMA).

A new type of CAR T cell is in development. Called allogeneic CAR T cells, they are formed from the blood of healthy donors or from umbilical cord blood.

Serious side effects

One of the most common, serious side effects of CAR T is cytokine release syndrome (CRS). It is the focus of Part 2. A range of problems affecting the brain and nervous system is also possible. Together this group of side effects is called neurotoxicity. Immune effector cell-associated neurotoxicity syndrome (ICANS) is a way to describe neurotoxicity caused by certain CAR T therapies. It is the focus of Part 3.

The U.S. FDA requires that makers of drugs or cell therapy products with very serious risks develop a Risk Evaluation and Mitigation Strategy (REMS). The purpose of a REMS is to ensure that the benefits of a drug outweigh its potential risks. It also ensures that providers are educated in treating CAR T side effects. All of the approved CAR T-cell therapies have a REMS.

The CAR T process

Immune cells are first taken from your blood. White blood cells called T cells are collected. The cells are sent to a lab. There they are modified by adding a gene to produce a receptor called chimeric antigen receptor (CAR). This is how CAR T cells are made.

Once the CAR T cells are made, they are allowed to multiply to achieve the required dose. Most people receive a short course of chemotherapy, after which the cells are put back into the bloodstream. CAR guides the T cells to find and kill cancer cells using a "search and destroy" approach. CAR T cells are one type of immune effector cell (IEC).

CAR T-cell therapy is both a gene therapy and an immunotherapy.

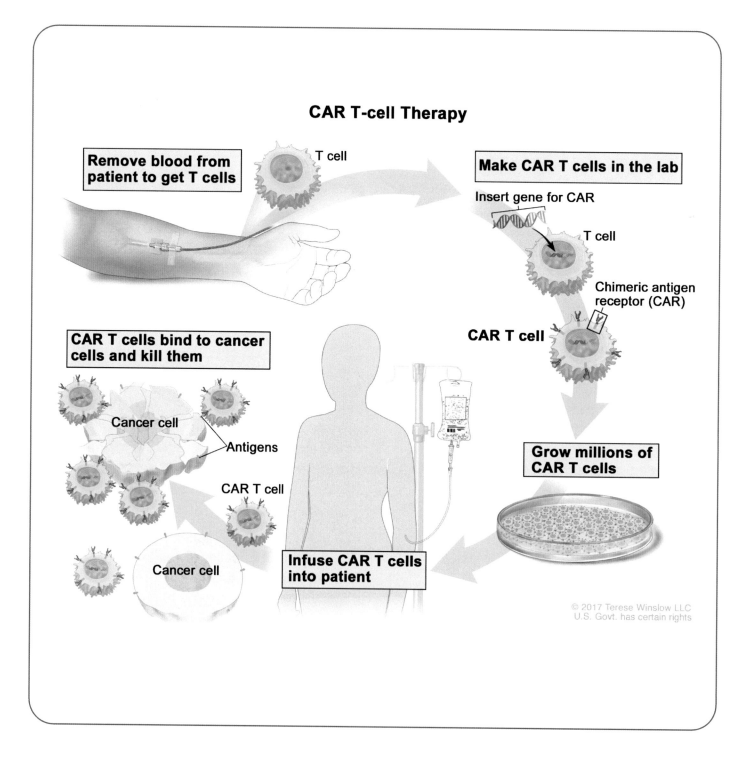

CAR T-cell Therapy

Remove blood from patient to get T cells

T cell

Make CAR T cells in the lab

Insert gene for CAR

T cell

Chimeric antigen receptor (CAR)

CAR T cell

CAR T cells bind to cancer cells and kill them

Cancer cell

Antigens

CAR T cell

Cancer cell

Infuse CAR T cells into patient

Grow millions of CAR T cells

© 2017 Terese Winslow LLC
U.S. Govt. has certain rights

Before and during infusion

Central venous access

CAR T products are given intravenously. This means they are put directly into the bloodstream through a vein. A type of catheter called a central venous catheter is often used when long-term (weeks or months) vein access is needed. A thin tube is inserted into your vein, usually below the collarbone or in the upper arm. The tube is guided into a large vein above the right side of the heart. When needed, this catheter will be accessed to draw blood, give fluids or medicines, or administer CAR T-cell therapy.

Heart check

CAR T-cell therapy can affect the heart. It can cause changes in heartbeat and other problems. Before receiving CAR T, your doctor will want to check your heart. This will provide a baseline (starting) picture of your heart's structure and function. A heart ultrasound (echocardiogram) is often ordered. This noninvasive test is performed using a hand-held wand placed on your chest. It does not use radiation. If you have a history of heart problems, your doctor will consult with a heart expert (cardiologist).

Neurologic (neuro) exam

CAR T-cell therapy can cause brain and nervous system problems. Expect to have a neurologic ("neuro") exam before receiving your cells. Neurologic means having to do with the nervous system. This check provides a point of comparison for testing done after infusion. The extent of the exam will vary between providers.

At a minimum, the exam will check your mental status. This is your level of awareness and ability to interact with your surroundings. The Immune Effector Cell-Associated

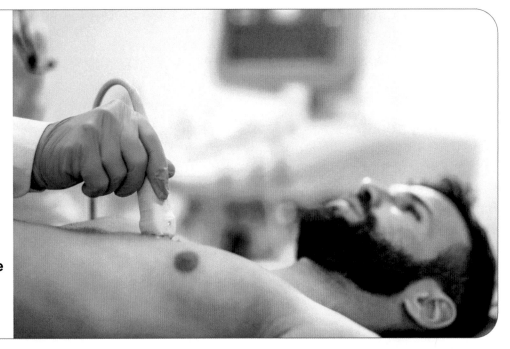

Echocardiogram

CAR T can cause heart problems. It is important for your doctor to know how your heart looks and works before you receive CAR T cells. An echocardiogram ("echo") is often ordered. It is a painless ultrasound of the heart.

Encephalopathy (ICE) Assessment Tool is often used. This screening test measures your ability to carry out simple tasks, such as writing and counting. Other tests and tools may be used to check your:

> Motor (movement) and sensory skills

> Balance and coordination

> Reflexes

> Nerve function

Your doctor may also order magnetic resonance imaging (MRI) of your brain. This can be helpful to compare with brain images taken if neurotoxicity develops after infusion.

Tumor lysis syndrome

Cancer cells break apart when they die. The contents of the dead cells enter the bloodstream. They disrupt the chemical balance of the blood. This is called tumor lysis syndrome (TLS). It is a serious side effect of cancer treatment. It can lead to organ damage and be life-threatening. TLS most often occurs after treatment of large tumors or fast-growing cancers. If this applies to your cancer, your doctor will take steps to prevent TLS. You will be monitored closely.

Preventing seizures

Some CAR T therapies are more likely to affect the brain than others. On the day of infusion, or anytime after, your doctor may start you on a medication to prevent seizures. A drug called levetiracetam is often given. It is an anti-convulsant. Anti-convulsants reduce abnormal overactivity in the brain. Levetiracetam is usually taken as a pill every 12 hours for up to 30 days.

After infusion

You might stay in the hospital for about a week after CAR T-cell therapy. This allows for close monitoring and treatment of urgent side effects. Early signs of CRS or nervous system problems will be easier to spot while being monitored in the hospital.

If hospital (inpatient) care is not needed, close monitoring by a center with CAR T experience may be an option. At the first sign of CRS or nervous system problems, hospitalization is needed.

You will have ongoing blood testing while in the hospital. Testing will look for any deficiencies or problems. Blood tests you are likely to have include:

> Complete blood count (CBC)

> Comprehensive metabolic panel (CMP)

> Blood clotting tests

> C-reactive protein (CRP)

> Ferritin (a protein that stores iron for the body to use)

After leaving the hospital you will continue to be closely monitored for side effects. Most patients are watched closely for about 4 weeks, or longer if needed. You will be instructed not to drive or do any other hazardous activities for at least 8 weeks after infusion.

Low blood cell counts

For weeks to months after CAR T-cell therapy your levels of red and white blood cells and platelets may be lower than normal. Low blood cell counts raise your risk of infection. One or both of the following may be used to try to lower the risk of infection:

> Blood and platelet transfusions

> Growth factors

Blood transfusions can raise the levels of red blood cells and/or platelets. In a transfusion, cells donated by healthy volunteers are put into your bloodstream through a vein.

Growth factors are medications that drive bone marrow to make more blood cells. They are given by injection or IV. Erythropoiesis-stimulating agents (ESAs) are growth factors that help the body make more red blood cells. Colony-stimulating growth factors such as filgrastim can also help your body make more white blood cells.

Low numbers of B cells

CAR T-cell therapy is most often used to treat B-cell non-Hodgkin lymphomas. In the process of killing cancer cells, normal B cells are also destroyed. A low level of B cells is called B-cell aplasia. It is a common side effect of CAR T. Depending on the type of CAR T received, it may last a long time. Having too few B cells is a good sign. It means that the CAR T cells continue to fight the cancer. But, it also means that you have fewer antibodies to protect you from infection.

Some people will have frequent infusions of a particular therapy called intravenous immunoglobulin therapy (IVIG). The antibodies used for the IVIG infusions come from different people. These donated antibodies help strengthen your immune system and fight infection. IVIG is typically only given if you are getting serious or repeated infections.

Key points

> CAR T-cell therapy is a type of immunotherapy. Immune cells are modified in a lab and put back in the body.

> The modified immune cells find and kill cancer cells using a "search and destroy" approach.

> Expect to stay at or close to the hospital after infusion. This allows for close monitoring and treatment of urgent side effects.

> You will be instructed not to drive or do any other hazardous activities for at least 8 weeks after infusion.

> Cytokine release syndrome (CRS) is one of the most common side effects of CAR T-cell therapy.

> Nervous system problems can occur after CAR T-cell therapy. Immune effector cell-associated neurotoxicity syndrome (ICANS) is one way to describe these side effects.

> Low blood cell counts are common after CAR T. You may receive blood transfusions and/or growth factors to help prevent infection.

> Having low numbers of B cells is called B-cell aplasia. It is a common, long-term side effect of CAR T therapy.

> Intravenous immunoglobulin (IVIG) may be used to strengthen your immune system and fight infection after CAR T-cell therapy.

2

Cytokine release syndrome (CRS)

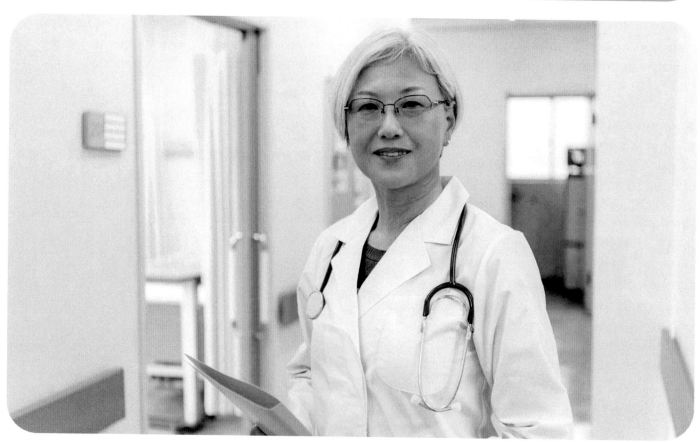

Cytokine release syndrome (CRS) is a common, serious side effect of CAR T-cell therapy. Although CRS is often mild, it can be severe.

What is CRS?

Cytokines are proteins. They carry out different immune-related jobs in the body. Some types cause inflammation. Other types help to reduce it.

In the days after a CAR T infusion, immune cells affected by the treatment may release many inflammation-causing cytokines into the blood. This causes your immune system to go into overdrive. A number of signs and symptoms are possible as a result. They include:

- Fever
- Low blood pressure
- Low tissue oxygen level
- Chills
- Rapid heartbeat
- Trouble breathing
- Nausea
- Rash
- Headache
- Muscle and joint aches

CRS usually starts 2 to 4 days after infusion and lasts about a week. However, it can start as early as hours after infusion and as late as 10 to 15 days afterward.

CRS can lead to damage to major organs. The heart, liver, kidneys, and/or lungs may be affected.

While most people experience CRS, you do not need it for CAR T to work. Your cancer type and the specific CAR T medicine you are treated with play a role in how likely you are to get CRS.

Serious CRS problems

CRS is mild for most people, but serious and possibly deadly problems are possible. These are described next.

Low blood pressure

Blood pressure is the strength of blood pushing against the sides of blood vessels. CRS can cause blood pressure to drop. Low blood pressure (hypotension) is dangerous. It reduces blood flow to the heart, brain, and other vital organs. In severe cases, low blood pressure can be life-threatening. Severely low blood pressure is treated with vasopressors. These medicines raise blood pressure by contracting (tightening) blood vessels.

Lack of oxygen to tissues

Hypoxia is a dangerous condition. It happens when there is not enough oxygen reaching the cells and tissues of the body. The brain, liver, and other organs can be damaged in minutes if they do not get enough oxygen.

Oxygen therapy is used to make sure that your tissues and organs are getting enough oxygen. Oxygen may be given through noninvasive nose tubes or a mask that covers your nose and mouth. The method used to give oxygen will depend on how low the level is.

In severe cases, intubation may be needed. Intubation refers to putting a tube through the mouth and into the airway. The tube is connected to a respirator that moves air in and out of your lungs. This is called mechanical ventilation.

Other serious problems

Effects on the heart
CRS can cause changes in the way the heart beats. It may beat faster, slower, or at abnormal intervals. Atrial fibrillation ("a-fib") refers to a fast and irregular heartbeat. In ventricular tachycardia ("V-tack") the heart beats quickly but regularly. Changes in heartbeat can be dangerous. Extra medications and treatment may be needed.

CRS can also cause your heart to not work as well. This is often temporary. While uncommon, the heart can also suddenly stop working after CAR T. This is called sudden cardiac arrest. It causes you to stop breathing and pass out.

Poor kidney function
The kidneys filter waste from the blood. CRS can cause the kidneys to stop working as they should. They suddenly stop filtering blood. This is called acute kidney injury (AKI). This is not common. If it occurs, the effects are often reversible (not permanent).

Capillary leak syndrome
This syndrome is a condition in which fluid and proteins leak out of the bloodstream. They leak out through tiny blood vessels (capillaries). It can lead to dangerously low blood pressure, organ failure, and shock. Shock is a life-threatening problem. It occurs when there is a sudden drop in blood flow in the body.

Macrophage activation syndrome (MAS)
A macrophage is a type of immune system cell. It kills viruses and bacteria and gets rid of dead cells. It also stimulates the action of other immune cells. MAS is a condition in which the body becomes flooded with "bad" cytokines. This can lead to organ damage. MAS can occur as part of CRS or on its own.

How severe is it?

Doctors use a grading system to assign CRS a grade from 1 (mildest) to 4 (most severe). The grade helps guide treatment decisions.

> **Grade 1** – Fever above 38 degrees Celsius (100.4 degrees Fahrenheit)

> **Grade 2** – Fever + slightly low blood pressure and/or slightly low oxygen level

> **Grade 3** – Fever + low blood pressure requiring 1 medication and/or moderately low oxygen level

> **Grade 4** – Fever + low blood pressure requiring more than one medication and/or severely low oxygen level

See the next page for treatment information.

Treatment

Tocilizumab (Actemra)

Interleukin-6 (IL-6) is a cytokine released during CRS. This leads to very high levels of it in the blood. Tocilizumab is a prescription medicine that blocks interaction between IL-6 and its receptors. It is given intravenously to treat CRS.

Tocilizumab is essential for treating moderate to severe CRS (grades 2, 3, and 4). It is also used to treat milder (grade 1) CRS in certain cases. It may be given for mild CRS lasting longer than 3 days (or less, depending on the specific CAR T therapy). It may also be given to treat mild CRS in the elderly, those with nervous system symptoms, and/or other health problems.

Steroids

Corticosteroids (steroids for short) are drugs that reduce the activity of the immune system. They are not the same as steroids used to build muscle mass (anabolic steroids). Intravenous steroids are used together with tocilizumab to treat more severe CRS, and sometimes milder CRS. They are also used to treat more severe neurologic side effects. Dexamethasone and methylprednisolone are commonly used steroids.

Key points

> CRS is the release of inflammation-causing cytokines into the blood after an infusion of CAR T-cell therapy.

> CRS happens to most people. It is the most common, serious side effect of CAR T-cell therapy.

> Although CRS is often mild, it can be severe.

> Signs and symptoms include fever, low blood pressure, low tissue oxygen, chills, rapid heartbeat, nausea, rash, headache, and trouble breathing.

> Other possible side effects of CRS include heart problems, acute kidney injury, capillary leak syndrome, and macrophage activation syndrome.

> Tocilizumab is a drug that blocks a cytokine released during CRS. It is essential for treating moderate to severe CRS.

> Steroids are used together with tocilizumab to treat moderate to severe CRS.

3
Nervous system side effects

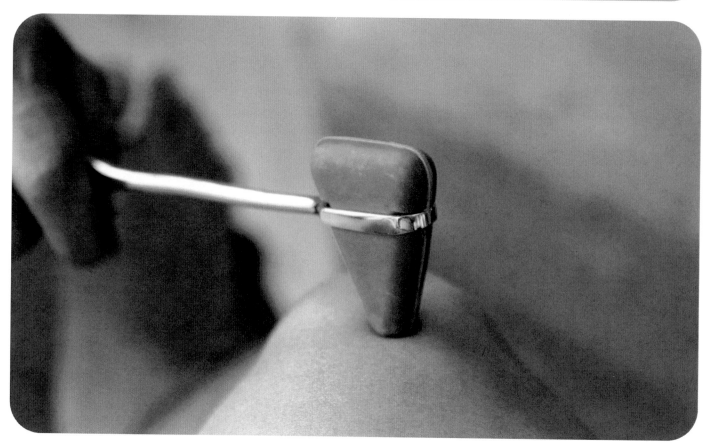

CAR T-cell therapy can cause brain and nervous system problems. While the most common symptoms are mild, very serious problems can occur. These side effects are usually reversible if treated promptly.

About nervous system effects

The brain, the spinal cord, and the nerves from these areas make up the nervous system. This complex system controls everything the body does. Movement, sensation, and breathing are all guided by the nervous system. It is the hub of all things mental including thought, memory, and learning.

Doctors call the nervous system side effects of immunotherapy "neurotoxicities." Immune effector cell-associated neurotoxicity syndrome (ICANS) is a term used to describe some but not all of these effects. Immune effector cell (IEC) is another term for a CAR T cell.

Common, mild symptoms include:

> Headache

> Dizziness

> Trouble sleeping

> Shaking

> Confusion

> Memory issues

> Anxiety

> Trouble finding words or speaking

In more severe cases, seizures, brain swelling, and coma can occur. These may be life-threatening. These and other possible symptoms are described below.

Nervous system side effects typically start 4 to 10 days after treatment. They tend to last about 2 weeks, but can last as long as 4 to 8 weeks.

Delirium
Delirium is a sudden change in brain function. It causes confusion, disorientation, and changes in behavior or emotions. It can also cause agitation, seeing things that aren't there (hallucinations), and extreme excitement. Delirium comes on quickly, often in a matter of hours to days.

Nerve problems
Your autonomic nervous system is always working behind the scenes. It regulates your basic body functions. This includes your heart rate, digestion, breathing rate, and body temperature. ICANS can cause this system to not work as well. This causes symptoms such as dizziness upon standing up, sweating too much or too little, and bowel and bladder problems.

Language problems
Aphasia is the loss of ability to understand or express speech. It is caused by injury to the brain. Aphasia is a language disorder–it does not affect intelligence. People with aphasia are still able to formulate thoughts in the same way. They are just unable to express them as they did before. This can be very frustrating.

Serious problems

The uncommon but serious nervous system side effects of CAR T-cell therapy are described next.

Seizures

Abnormal electrical signals in the brain can cause sudden and uncontrolled body movements. Shaking in particular is common. These are called seizures. Other symptoms include behavior changes, loss of awareness, and loss of muscle control.

Convulsive status epilepticus is the medical term for having one long (5 minutes or more) seizure, or several shorter seizures in a row. Convulsive status epilepticus is a medical emergency that can occur in severe ICANS. Hospital treatment typically includes use of several different types of drugs. They are given in a specific order.

Brain swelling

Swelling due to trapped fluid is the body's response to many types of injury and illness. Swelling of the brain is a life-threatening reaction to CAR T. When the brain swells, it increases the pressure inside the skull.

Medicines are used to draw fluid out of the skull and injured brain. This is called osmotic therapy or hyperosmolar therapy. In severe cases of brain swelling, a lumbar puncture (described on the next page) or ventriculostomy may be needed. Ventriculostomy is a procedure that involves inserting a plastic tube into the skull. Excess fluid drains through the tube in order to lower the pressure.

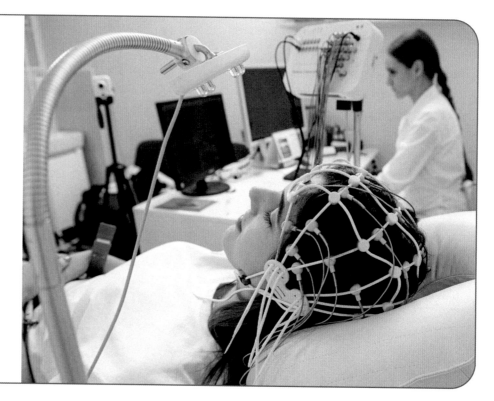

Monitoring for seizures

You may have electroencephalography (EEG) to monitor for seizures during ICANS. An EEG is a recording of electrical activity in the brain.

Assessment and supportive care

Testing and care you may have while in the hospital are described next.

Neurologic exams
You will have frequent neurologic exams while in the hospital. These check your mental status and motor function. They also look for other signs of brain and nervous system problems.

Supportive care
You may receive fluids intravenously (an "IV drip") to keep you hydrated. Your care team will also take steps to prevent food or liquid from going into your airway instead of your food pipe (esophagus). Food or fluids in the airway is called aspiration. It can lead to infection (often pneumonia) and inflamed lungs.

Monitoring for seizures
You may be monitored for seizures. An electroencephalogram (EEG) is used. An EEG is a recording of electrical activity in the brain. It tracks and records brain wave patterns. The patterns are relayed by small metal sensors placed on your scalp.

Brain imaging
You may have magnetic resonance imaging (MRI) of your brain to look for swelling or damage. If MRI is not possible, you may have computed tomography (CT) instead.

Lumbar puncture
A lumbar puncture may be needed for more severe ICANS. The fluid that flows in and around the brain and spinal cord is called cerebrospinal fluid (CSF). Lumbar puncture is a simple bedside procedure to remove a sample of spinal fluid for testing. It can also

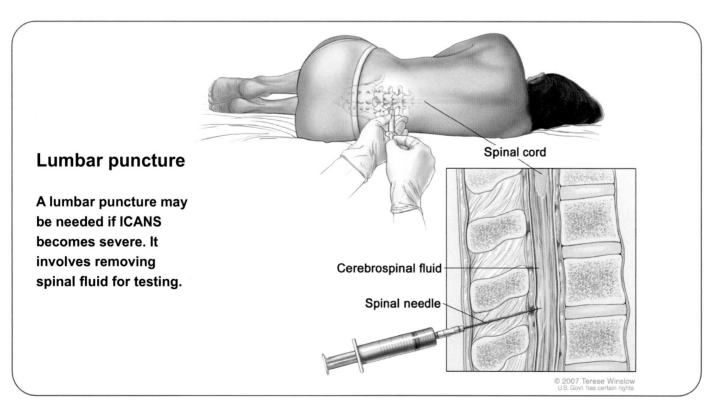

Lumbar puncture

A lumbar puncture may be needed if ICANS becomes severe. It involves removing spinal fluid for testing.

Spinal cord

Cerebrospinal fluid

Spinal needle

© 2007 Terese Winslow
U.S. Govt. has certain rights

be used to measure and relieve pressure from brain swelling.

How severe is it?

Doctors use a point system to assign ICANS a grade from 1 to 4. A score of 4 is the most severe (life threatening). The grade helps guide treatment decisions.

One key factor in the overall grade is the Immune Effector Cell-Associated Encephalopathy (ICE) score. The ICE Assessment Tool is an ICANS screening test. It provides a snapshot of your mental state. It measures your ability to carry out simple tasks, such as writing and counting. A score of 0 (critical emergency) to 10 (mild) is possible.

In addition to ICE score, the following information helps determine the overall severity of ICANS:

> How alert/responsive you are

> Whether you are having seizures

> Whether you have severe muscle weakness

> Whether there is brain swelling

The ICANS grading system was developed by the American Society of Blood and Marrow Transplantation, now the American Society for Transplantation and Cellular Therapy (ASTCT).

Treatment

For mild ICANS, supportive care is often all that is needed. Moderate or severe ICANS is treated with steroids given through a vein. Steroids are medicines that reduce immune system activity. They relieve inflammation in the body. Dexamethasone and methylprednisolone are widely used steroids.

Those with both ICANS (any grade) and cytokine release syndrome (CRS) will also be given tocilizumab. See page 15 for more information on tocilizumab.

Key points

- The nervous system side effects of CAR T-cell therapy are called neurotoxicities.

- They include immune effector cell-associated neurotoxicity syndrome (ICANS) and some other symptoms.

- Common symptoms include headache, delirium, dizziness, trouble sleeping, shaking, and anxiety.

- Language and nerve problems are also possible.

- Very serious nervous system effects include seizures, brain swelling, and coma. These are usually reversible.

- Supportive care may be all that is needed for mild nervous system side effects.

- Intravenous steroids are used to treat moderate to severe ICANS.

- Tocilizumab is given as an added single-dose therapy for people with both ICANS and cytokine release syndrome.

Let us know what you think!

Please take a moment to complete an online survey about the NCCN Guidelines for Patients.

NCCN.org/patients/response

4
Resources

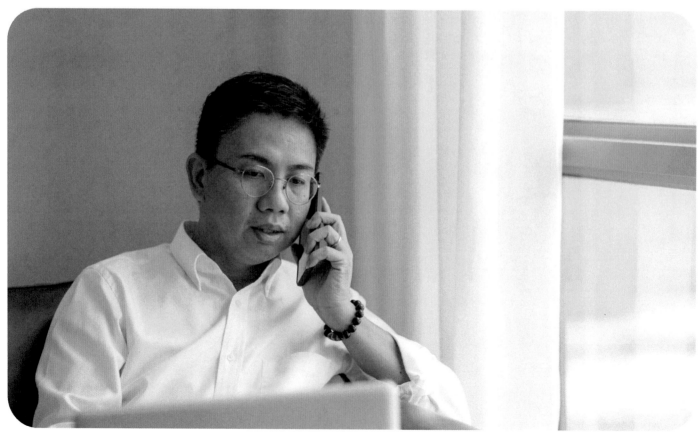

CAR T-cell therapy is a recent innovation in cancer treatment. This chapter includes resources for learning more about this type of immunotherapy and its effects.

Questions to ask your doctor

It is normal to have lots of questions about immunotherapy with CAR T-cell therapy. Possible questions to ask your doctor are listed on the following pages. Feel free to use these questions or come up with your own.

Following the questions is a listing of websites that provide information for patients about CAR T-cell therapy and its effects.

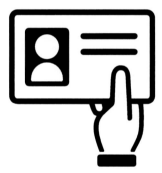

Immunotherapy Wallet Card

Ask your doctor for an immunotherapy wallet card. This card states that you have received CAR T-cell therapy. It also lists potential side effects and contact numbers for your cancer care team. Carry it with you at all times. If a card is not available, ask for a printable list of your treatment regimen. A printable card is also available in the *Resources* section of this patient guide (see page 25).

Questions to ask your doctor about CAR T side effects

1. What are the most common side effects of CAR T-cell therapy?

2. Are any of the side effects permanent?

3. When do they start? How long do they usually last?

4. How are they treated?

5. I didn't experience cytokine release syndrome (CRS). Is that bad?

6. How soon can I resume my normal activities after receiving CAR T-cell therapy?

7. How severe are my symptoms?

8. Are there any known long-term side effects of CAR T?

9. After I leave the hospital, which symptoms should I report right away? How do I report them?

10. Can I report symptoms or communicate with my treatment team online?

11. Can you give me an immunotherapy wallet card?

Websites

American Cancer Society
cancer.org/treatment/treatments-and-side-effects/treatment-types/immunotherapy/car-t-cell1.html

Be the Match
BeTheMatch.org

CancerCare
cancercare.org

Cancer Support Community
cancersupportcommunity.org

Good Days
mygooddays.org

Leukaemia Care
leukaemiacare.org.uk/support-and-information/latest-from-leukaemia-care/blog/cart-t-therapy

Lymphoma Research Foundation
lymphoma.org/aboutlymphoma/treatments/cartcell

National Coalition for Cancer Survivorship
canceradvocacy.org

Oncology Nursing Society
Immunotherapy Wallet Cards
ons.org

PAN Foundation
panfoundation.org

Stupid Cancer
stupidcancer.org

The Leukemia & Lymphoma Society
www.LLS.org/CartTherapy

LLS Clinical Trial Support Center
www.LLS.org/CTSC

U.S. National Library of Medicine Clinical Trials Database
clinicaltrials.gov

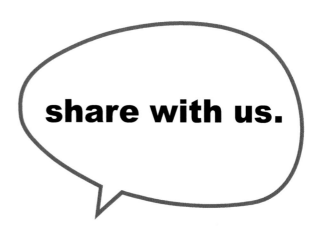

share with us.

Take our survey
And help make the
NCCN Guidelines for Patients
better for everyone!

NCCN.org/patients/comments

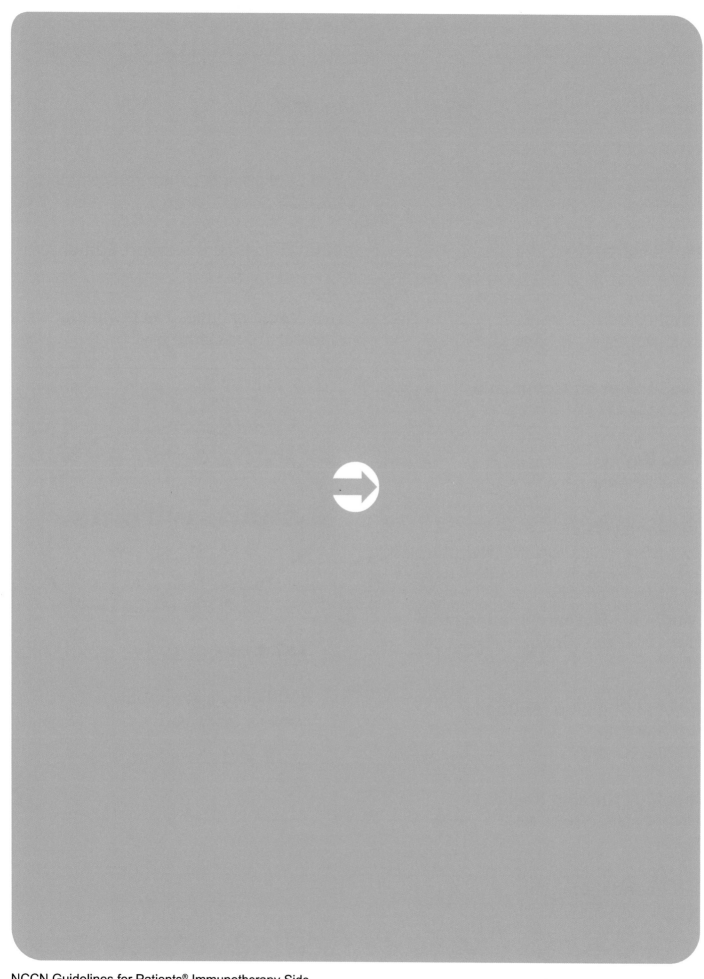

Words to know

aphasia
A language disorder caused by injury to the brain. A possible neurologic side effect of CAR T-cell therapy.

B-cell aplasia
Having low numbers of B cells. A common and sometimes long-term side effect of CAR T-cell therapy.

capillary leak syndrome
The escape of fluid and proteins from blood vessels into surrounding tissues. Results in dangerously low blood pressure.

cerebral edema
Brain swelling that causes an increase in pressure inside the skull. A possible side effect of CAR T-cell therapy.

chimeric antigen receptor (CAR) T-cell therapy
A type of immunotherapy in which T cells (a type of immune system cell) are modified in a way that allows them to find and kill cancer cells.

convulsive status epilepticus
A seizure lasting longer than 5 minutes, or having multiple seizures within a 5-minute period without fully recovering between them.

corticosteroids
Inflammation-reducing medicines. They reduce the activity of the immune system. Used to treat side effects of CAR T-cell therapy.

cytokine release syndrome (CRS)
A potentially serious side effect of CAR T-cell therapy. Caused by the release of inflammatory proteins into the blood from immune cells affected by the immunotherapy.

delirium
A mental state causing confusion, disorientation, and memory problems. May also cause agitation, hallucinations, and extreme excitement. A possible side effect of CAR T-cell therapy.

hypogammaglobulinemia
An immune system problem in which not enough antibodies are made, resulting in increased infection risk.

hypotension
Low blood pressure. A possible complication of cytokine release syndrome.

hypoxia
Decreased oxygen reaching body tissue. A possible complication of cytokine release syndrome.

immune effector cell-associated neurotoxicity syndrome (ICANS)
A group of nervous system-related side effects of CAR T-cell therapy.

intravenous immunoglobulin (IVIG)
A solution made from antibodies taken from the blood of healthy donors is given through a vein. Sometimes given to prevent infections after CAR T.

macrophage activation syndrome (MAS)
A serious problem in which too many of a type of white blood cell and T cells are made by the body. A possible complication of CRS.

osmotic therapy
The use of medicines to draw fluid out of the skull and the brain, reducing pressure. Also called hyperosmolar therapy.

Risk Evaluation and Mitigation Strategy (REMS)
A strategy to ensure that the benefits of using a drug outweigh its serious potential

risks. Required by the U.S. Food & Drug Administration (FDA) for currently available CAR T-cell therapies.

seizure
Sudden, uncontrolled body movements and changes in behavior caused by abnormal electrical activity in the brain.

tocilizumab (Actemra)
A prescription medicine used to treat severe or life-threatening cytokine release syndrome caused by CAR T-cell therapy.

tumor lysis syndrome (TLS)
A problem caused by treatment of large or fast-growing cancers. The contents of dead cancer cells are released into the blood. This causes problems and may cause organ damage.

vasopressor
Medicine that raises blood pressure by contracting (tightening) blood vessels. Used in emergency situations to treat severely low blood pressure.

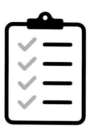

We want your feedback!

Our goal is to provide helpful and easy-to-understand information on cancer.

Take our survey to let us know what we got right and what we could do better:

NCCN.org/patients/feedback

Notes

NCCN Cancer Centers

Abramson Cancer Center
at the University of Pennsylvania
Philadelphia, Pennsylvania
800.789.7366 • pennmedicine.org/cancer

Case Comprehensive Cancer Center/
University Hospitals Seidman Cancer
Center and Cleveland Clinic Taussig
Cancer Institute
Cleveland, Ohio
800.641.2422 • UH Seidman Cancer Center
uhhospitals.org/services/cancer-services
866.223.8100 • CC Taussig Cancer Institute
my.clevelandclinic.org/departments/cancer
216.844.8797 • Case CCC
case.edu/cancer

City of Hope National Medical Center
Los Angeles, California
800.826.4673 • cityofhope.org

Dana-Farber/Brigham and Women's
Cancer Center | Massachusetts General
Hospital Cancer Center
Boston, Massachusetts
617.732.5500 • youhaveus.org
617.726.5130
massgeneral.org/cancer-center

Duke Cancer Institute
Durham, North Carolina
888.275.3853 • dukecancerinstitute.org

Fox Chase Cancer Center
Philadelphia, Pennsylvania
888.369.2427 • foxchase.org

Fred & Pamela Buffett Cancer Center
Omaha, Nebraska
402.559.5600 • unmc.edu/cancercenter

Fred Hutchinson Cancer
Research Center/Seattle
Cancer Care Alliance
Seattle, Washington
206.606.7222 • seattlecca.org
206.667.5000 • fredhutch.org

Huntsman Cancer Institute
at the University of Utah
Salt Lake City, Utah
800.824.2073 • huntsmancancer.org

Indiana University
Melvin and Bren Simon
Comprehensive Cancer Center
Indianapolis, Indiana
888.600.4822 • www.cancer.iu.edu

Mayo Clinic Cancer Center
Phoenix/Scottsdale, Arizona
Jacksonville, Florida
Rochester, Minnesota
480.301.8000 • Arizona
904.953.0853 • Florida
507.538.3270 • Minnesota
mayoclinic.org/cancercenter

Memorial Sloan Kettering
Cancer Center
New York, New York
800.525.2225 • mskcc.org

Moffitt Cancer Center
Tampa, Florida
888.663.3488 • moffitt.org

O'Neal Comprehensive
Cancer Center at UAB
Birmingham, Alabama
800.822.0933 • uab.edu/onealcancercenter

Robert H. Lurie Comprehensive Cancer
Center of Northwestern University
Chicago, Illinois
866.587.4322 • cancer.northwestern.edu

Roswell Park Comprehensive
Cancer Center
Buffalo, New York
877.275.7724 • roswellpark.org

Siteman Cancer Center at Barnes-
Jewish Hospital and Washington
University School of Medicine
St. Louis, Missouri
800.600.3606 • siteman.wustl.edu

St. Jude Children's
Research Hospital/
The University of Tennessee
Health Science Center
Memphis, Tennessee
866.278.5833 • stjude.org
901.448.5500 • uthsc.edu

Stanford Cancer Institute
Stanford, California
877.668.7535 • cancer.stanford.edu

The Ohio State University
Comprehensive Cancer Center -
James Cancer Hospital and
Solove Research Institute
Columbus, Ohio
800.293.5066 • cancer.osu.edu

The Sidney Kimmel Comprehensive
Cancer Center at Johns Hopkins
Baltimore, Maryland
410.955.8964
www.hopkinskimmelcancercenter.org

The University of Texas
MD Anderson Cancer Center
Houston, Texas
844.269.5922 • mdanderson.org

UC Davis
Comprehensive Cancer Center
Sacramento, California
916.734.5959 • 800.770.9261
health.ucdavis.edu/cancer

UC San Diego Moores Cancer Center
La Jolla, California
858.822.6100 • cancer.ucsd.edu

UCLA Jonsson
Comprehensive Cancer Center
Los Angeles, California
310.825.5268 • cancer.ucla.edu

UCSF Helen Diller Family
Comprehensive Cancer Center
San Francisco, California
800.689.8273 • cancer.ucsf.edu

University of Colorado Cancer Center
Aurora, Colorado
720.848.0300 • coloradocancercenter.org

University of Michigan
Rogel Cancer Center
Ann Arbor, Michigan
800.865.1125 • rogelcancercenter.org

University of Wisconsin
Carbone Cancer Center
Madison, Wisconsin
608.265.1700 • uwhealth.org/cancer

UT Southwestern Simmons
Comprehensive Cancer Center
Dallas, Texas
214.648.3111 • utsouthwestern.edu/simmons

Vanderbilt-Ingram Cancer Center
Nashville, Tennessee
877.936.8422 • vicc.org

Yale Cancer Center/
Smilow Cancer Hospital
New Haven, Connecticut
855.4.SMILOW • yalecancercenter.org

NCCN Contributors

This patient guide is based on the NCCN Clinical Practice Guidelines in Oncology (NCCN Guidelines®) for Management of Immunotherapy-Related Toxicities, Version 1.2022. It was adapted, reviewed, and published with help from the following people:

Dorothy A. Shead, MS
Senior Director
Patient Information Operations

Erin Vidic, MA
Medical Writer

Susan Kidney
Senior Graphic Design Specialist

The NCCN Clinical Practice Guidelines in Oncology (NCCN Guidelines®) for Management of Immunotherapy-Related Toxicities, Version 1.2022 were developed by the following NCCN Panel Members:

John A. Thompson, MD/Chair
Fred Hutchinson Cancer Research Center/
Seattle Cancer Care Alliance

Bryan J. Schneider, MD/Vice-Chair
University of Michigan Rogel Cancer Center

Julie Brahmer, MD/Vice-Chair
The Sidney Kimmel Comprehensive
Cancer Center at Johns Hopkins

Amaka Achufusi, MD
University of Wisconsin
Carbone Cancer Center

*Philippe Armand, MD, PhD
Dana-Farber/Brigham and Women's
Cancer Center | Massachusetts General
Hospital Cancer Center

Meghan K. Berkenstock, MD
The Sidney Kimmel Comprehensive
Cancer Center at Johns Hopkins

Shailender Bhatia, MD
Fred Hutchinson Cancer Research Center/
Seattle Cancer Care Alliance

*Lihua E. Budde, MD, PhD
City of Hope National Medical Center

Saurin Chokshi, MD
St. Jude Children's Research Hospital/
The University of Tennessee
Health Science Center

Marianne Davies, DNP, RN, AOCNP
Yale Cancer Center/Smilow Cancer Hospital

Amro Elshoury, MD
Roswell Park Comprehensive Cancer Cente

Yaron Gesthalter, MD
UCSF Helen Diller Family
Comprehensive Cancer Center

Aparna Hegde, MD
O'Neal Comprehensive
Cancer Center at UAB

Michael Jain, MD, PhD
Moffitt Cancer Center

Benjamin H. Kaffenberger
The Ohio State University Comprehensive
Cancer Center - James Cancer Hospital
and Solove Research Institute

Melissa G. Lechner, MD, PhD
UCLA Jonsson
Comprehensive Cancer Center

Tianhong Li, MD, PhD
UC Davis Comprehensive Cancer Center

Alissa Marr, MD
Fred & Pamela Buffett Cancer Center

Suzanne McGettigan, MSN, CRNP
Abramson Cancer Center
at the University of Pennsylvania

Jordan McPherson, PharmD, MS, BCOP
Huntsman Cancer Institute
at the University of Utah

Theresa Medina, MD
University of Colorado Cancer Center

Nisha A. Mohindra, MD
Robert H. Lurie Comprehensive Cancer
Center of Northwestern University

Anthony J. Olszanski, MD, RPh
Fox Chase Cancer Center

*Olalekan Oluwole, MD
Vanderbilt-Ingram Cancer Center

Sandip P. Patel, MD
UC San Diego Moores Cancer Center

Pradnya Patil, MD
Case Comprehensive Cancer Center/
University Hospitals Seidman Cancer
Center and Cleveland Clinic Taussig
Cancer Institute

Sunil Reddy, MD
Stanford Cancer Institute

Mabel Ryder, MD
Mayo Clinic Cancer Center

*Bianca Santomasso, MD, PhD
Memorial Sloan Kettering Cancer Center

Scott Shofer, MD, PhD
Duke Cancer Institute

Jeffrey A. Sosman, MD
Robert H. Lurie Comprehensive Cancer
Center of Northwestern University

Yinghong Wang, MD, PhD
The University of Texas
MD Anderson Cancer Center

Vlad G. Zaha, MD, PhD
UT Southwestern Simmons
Comprehensive Cancer Center

NCCN Staff

Lisa Hang, PhD
Oncology Scientist/Medical Writer

Mary Dwyer, MS
Director, Guidelines Operations

Megan Lyons, MS
Guidelines Layout Specialist

* Reviewed this patient guide. For disclosures, visit NCCN.org/disclosures.

NCCN Guidelines for Patients® Immunotherapy Side
Effects: CAR T-Cell Therapy, 2022

Index

Made in the USA
Middletown, DE
24 April 2023

29410368R00020